Nature's Apothecary Quick Reference Guide to Oral Antibiotics

Luna Parnell

Table of Content

Introduction

Welcome to "Nature's Apothecary: Quick Reference Guide to Oral Antibiotics," a comprehensive exploration into the world of natural remedies for internal bacterial infections. As we continue our journey through the vast landscape of medicinal herbs, this section focuses on those that can be ingested to combat and prevent infections from the inside out. Drawing on centuries of traditional knowledge and supported by modern scientific research, these herbs offer powerful antibacterial properties that can help address a range of internal health issues.

In this guide, you will find detailed descriptions of various herbs renowned for their oral antibiotic properties. Each herb is explored in depth, providing you with an understanding of its scientific benefits, mechanisms of action, and the types of infections it can effectively target. We will delve into the dosages and preparations, offering easy-to-follow recipes to maximize the therapeutic potential of these natural remedies.

From gastrointestinal and respiratory infections to urinary tract infections, the herbs covered in this guide offer a natural, holistic approach to health and wellness. Our goal is to empower you with knowledge and practical applications that can be seamlessly integrated into your daily routine.

Join us as we uncover the power of nature's pharmacy and discover how these remarkable plants can support your body's defenses, promote healing, and enhance your overall well-being.

Ginger (Zingiber officinale)

Description: Ginger, scientifically known as Zingiber officinale, is a flowering plant whose rhizome, commonly referred to as ginger root, is widely used as a spice and for its medicinal properties. Originating from Southeast Asia, ginger has been an integral part of traditional medicine systems such as Ayurveda, Traditional Chinese Medicine, and herbal medicine in many cultures. It is known for its distinctive spicy and aromatic flavor.

Scientific Benefits: Ginger contains a variety of bioactive compounds, with gingerols and shogaols being the most prominent. These compounds contribute to ginger's powerful anti-inflammatory, antioxidant, and digestive-enhancing properties. Ginger is renowned for its ability to reduce nausea, improve digestion, and provide relief from colds and flu. It also supports cardiovascular health and has been shown to reduce pain and inflammation.

Antibacterial Properties: Ginger exhibits significant antibacterial activity, particularly against pathogens like Escherichia coli, Staphylococcus aureus, and Salmonella. The antibacterial properties of ginger are largely attributed to its bioactive compounds, which help inhibit the growth of harmful bacteria and support a healthy digestive system.

Types of Infections Targeted: Ginger is beneficial for treating and preventing various internal infections and conditions:

- **Digestive Health:** Ginger helps combat gastrointestinal infections, reduce nausea, and alleviate symptoms of indigestion and bloating.
- **Respiratory Health:** Its antimicrobial properties are effective in treating respiratory infections such as colds, sore throats, and bronchitis.
- **General Immunity:** Ginger supports overall immune function, helping the body to fight off infections more efficiently.

Dosage Recommendations: For oral use, ginger can be consumed in various forms, including fresh, dried, powdered, as a tea, or in supplement form. Generally, 1-3 grams of ginger per day is recommended for most therapeutic purposes. However, it is best to consult with a healthcare provider for personalized dosage recommendations.

Preparation Recipe: *Ginger Tea:*

1. **Ingredients:**
   - 1-2 inches fresh ginger root
   - 2 cups water
   - Honey or lemon (optional, for taste)
2. **Preparation:**
   - Peel the ginger root and slice it thinly.
   - Bring the water to a boil in a saucepan.
   - Add the sliced ginger to the boiling water.
   - Reduce the heat and let it simmer for 10-15 minutes.
   - Strain the tea into a cup.
3. **Serving:**
   - Add honey or lemon to taste, if desired.
   - Enjoy the tea warm to benefit from its soothing and antibacterial properties.

Turmeric (Curcuma longa)

Description: Turmeric, scientifically known as Curcuma longa, is a perennial herbaceous plant from the ginger family, Zingiberaceae. Native to Southeast Asia, particularly India, turmeric is characterized by its bright yellow-orange rhizome, which is widely used as a spice, dye, and medicinal herb. Turmeric has a long history of use in Ayurvedic and traditional Chinese medicine for its numerous health benefits.

Scientific Benefits: Turmeric is rich in bioactive compounds, the most notable being curcumin, which accounts for its vibrant color and therapeutic properties. Curcumin has been extensively studied for its potent anti-inflammatory, antioxidant, and antimicrobial effects. Turmeric is known to support digestive health, reduce inflammation, enhance immune function, and provide relief from various chronic conditions such as arthritis and cardiovascular diseases.

Antibacterial Properties: Turmeric exhibits significant antibacterial activity against a broad spectrum of bacteria, including both Gram-positive and Gram-negative strains. Curcumin, in particular, has been shown to inhibit the growth of pathogenic bacteria such as Staphylococcus aureus, Escherichia coli, and Salmonella typhi. Turmeric's antibacterial properties help in preventing and treating infections, promoting overall health and well-being.

Types of Infections Targeted: Turmeric is beneficial for treating and preventing various internal infections and conditions:

- **Digestive Health:** Turmeric aids in combating gastrointestinal infections, reducing symptoms of indigestion, bloating, and gas, and supporting gut health.
- **Respiratory Health:** Its antimicrobial properties are effective in treating respiratory infections such as colds, flu, and bronchitis.
- **General Immunity:** Turmeric enhances immune function, helping the body to fight off infections more effectively.

Dosage Recommendations: For oral use, turmeric can be consumed in various forms, including fresh, dried, powdered, as a tea, or in supplement form. Generally, 500-2000 mg of turmeric per day is recommended for most therapeutic purposes, with a curcumin content of 95%. However, it is best to consult with a healthcare provider for personalized dosage recommendations.

Preparation Recipe: *Golden Milk:*

1. **Ingredients:**
   - 1 cup milk (dairy or plant-based)
   - 1/2 teaspoon turmeric powder
   - 1/4 teaspoon ground ginger
   - 1/4 teaspoon ground cinnamon
   - 1 tablespoon honey or maple syrup (optional, for taste)
   - Pinch of black pepper (to enhance curcumin absorption)
2. **Preparation:**
   - In a small saucepan, combine the milk, turmeric powder, ground ginger, and ground cinnamon.
   - Heat the mixture over medium heat, stirring constantly until it is hot but not boiling.
   - Remove from heat and let it cool slightly.
3. **Serving:**
   - Add honey or maple syrup to taste, if desired.
   - Stir in a pinch of black pepper to enhance curcumin absorption.

Oregano (Origanum vulgare)

Description: Oregano, scientifically known as Origanum vulgare, is a perennial herb from the mint family, Lamiaceae. Native to the Mediterranean region, oregano is widely recognized for its aromatic, slightly bitter leaves and is commonly used as a culinary herb. Beyond its culinary uses, oregano has a rich history of medicinal applications, particularly for its potent antibacterial properties.

Antibiotic Properties: Oregano is known for its strong antibacterial activity, which is primarily attributed to its high content of phenolic compounds, such as carvacrol and thymol. These compounds have been shown to disrupt the cell membranes of bacteria, inhibiting their growth and reducing the risk of infection. Studies have demonstrated that oregano oil can be effective against a wide range of bacteria, including Escherichia coli, Staphylococcus aureus, and Pseudomonas aeruginosa.

Types of Infections Targeted: Oregano is particularly effective in treating and preventing various internal infections:

- **Respiratory Infections:** Oregano can help combat bacterial infections in the respiratory tract, such as bronchitis, sinusitis, and sore throats.
- **Digestive Infections:** Its antimicrobial properties are beneficial for addressing bacterial overgrowth in the gut, reducing symptoms of indigestion, bloating, and gastrointestinal discomfort.
- **Urinary Tract Infections:** Oregano can aid in treating and preventing urinary tract infections by inhibiting the growth of pathogenic bacteria.

Dosage Recommendations: For oral use, oregano can be consumed in various forms, including fresh or dried leaves, essential oil, or as a supplement. Generally, 100-200 mg of oregano oil (standardized to 60-80% carvacrol) per day is recommended for most therapeutic purposes. It is important to dilute oregano oil properly before ingestion and to consult with a healthcare provider for personalized dosage recommendations.

Preparation Recipe: *Oregano Infused Olive Oil:*

1. **Ingredients:**

- 1 cup extra virgin olive oil
- 1/4 cup dried oregano leaves
- 1-2 garlic cloves (optional, for additional antibacterial benefits)

2. **Preparation:**
   - Slightly crush the dried oregano leaves to release their essential oils.
   - Peel and lightly crush the garlic cloves.
   - Combine the olive oil, oregano leaves, and garlic cloves in a small saucepan.
   - Heat the mixture over low heat for 10-15 minutes, ensuring the oil does not boil.
   - Remove from heat and let it cool completely.

3. **Serving:**
   - Strain the oil through a fine-mesh sieve or cheesecloth into a clean, sterilized jar.
   - Store the infused oil in a cool, dark place.
   - Use the oregano-infused olive oil as a salad dressing, drizzle over cooked vegetables, or take a teaspoon daily to benefit from its antibacterial properties.

Thyme (Thymus vulgaris)

Description: Thyme, scientifically known as Thymus vulgaris, is a perennial herb belonging to the mint family, Lamiaceae. Native to the Mediterranean region, thyme is characterized by its small, aromatic leaves and purple or pink flowers. It has been used for centuries in culinary and medicinal applications, valued for its robust flavor and potent health benefits.

Antibiotic Properties: Thyme is renowned for its strong antibacterial activity, primarily due to its high content of essential oils, particularly thymol and carvacrol. These compounds have been extensively studied for their ability to disrupt the cell membranes of bacteria, leading to the inhibition of bacterial growth and the prevention of infection. Thyme has demonstrated effectiveness against a variety of pathogenic bacteria, including Staphylococcus aureus, Escherichia coli, and Helicobacter pylori.

Types of Infections Targeted: Thyme is effective in treating and preventing several internal infections:

- **Respiratory Infections:** Thyme helps combat bacterial infections in the respiratory system, such as bronchitis, pharyngitis, and tonsillitis. Its expectorant properties also aid in relieving congestion and cough.

- **Digestive Infections:** Thyme's antibacterial effects are beneficial for treating gastrointestinal infections, reducing symptoms of indigestion, gas, and bloating.
- **Oral Infections:** Thyme can help prevent and treat oral infections, including gingivitis, bad breath, and throat infections.

Dosage Recommendations: For oral use, thyme can be consumed in various forms, including fresh or dried leaves, as a tea, or in essential oil form. Generally, 1-2 grams of dried thyme leaves per day is recommended, or 2-4 drops of thyme essential oil diluted in a carrier oil. It is important to use thyme essential oil with caution and consult a healthcare provider for personalized dosage recommendations.

Preparation Recipe: *Thyme Tea:*

1. **Ingredients:**
    - 1-2 teaspoons dried thyme leaves (or 2-3 fresh sprigs)
    - 1 cup boiling water

- o Honey or lemon (optional, for taste)

2. **Preparation:**
   - o Place the dried thyme leaves or fresh sprigs in a tea infuser or teapot.
   - o Pour the boiling water over the thyme.
   - o Cover and let it steep for 5-10 minutes.
   - o Strain the tea into a cup.

3. **Serving:**
   - o Add honey or lemon to taste, if desired.
   - o Enjoy the tea warm to benefit from its soothing and antibacterial properties.

Neem (Azadirachta indica)

Description: Neem, scientifically known as Azadirachta indica, is a fast-growing tree native to the Indian subcontinent and widely found in tropical and subtropical regions. The neem tree has been a cornerstone of Ayurvedic medicine for centuries, revered for its extensive range of medicinal properties. Every part of the neem tree, including its leaves, bark, seeds, and oil, has therapeutic benefits, making it a versatile natural remedy.

Antibiotic Properties: Neem is known for its potent antibacterial properties, primarily attributed to compounds such as azadirachtin, nimbidin, and nimbin. These bioactive constituents have been shown to inhibit the growth of various pathogenic bacteria by disrupting their cell membranes and metabolic pathways. Neem exhibits broad-spectrum antibacterial activity against both Gram-positive and Gram-negative bacteria, including Escherichia coli, Staphylococcus aureus, and Streptococcus mutans.

Types of Infections Targeted: Neem is effective in treating and preventing several internal infections:

- **Digestive Infections:** Neem helps combat bacterial infections in the gastrointestinal tract, reducing symptoms of indigestion, diarrhea, and stomach ulcers.
- **Respiratory Infections:** Its antibacterial properties are beneficial for treating respiratory infections such as bronchitis, colds, and sore throats.
- **Oral Infections:** Neem is highly effective in maintaining oral hygiene, preventing and treating infections such as gingivitis, periodontitis, and bad breath.

Dosage Recommendations: For oral use, neem can be consumed in various forms, including fresh or dried leaves, neem leaf powder, or neem oil. Generally, 1-2 grams of neem leaf powder per day is recommended, or 1-2 drops of neem oil diluted in a carrier oil. It is crucial to use neem oil with caution and consult a healthcare provider for personalized dosage recommendations.

Preparation Recipe: *Neem Leaf Tea:*

1. **Ingredients:**
    - 1 teaspoon dried neem leaves (or 5-6 fresh neem leaves)

- o   2 cups water
- o   Honey or lemon (optional, for taste)

2. **Preparation:**
- o   Bring the water to a boil in a saucepan.
- o   Add the dried neem leaves or fresh neem leaves to the boiling water.
- o   Reduce the heat and let it simmer for 10-15 minutes.
- o   Strain the tea into a cup.

3. **Serving:**
- o   Add honey or lemon to taste, if desired.
- o   Consume the tea warm to benefit from its antibacterial and therapeutic properties.

Cloves (Syzygium aromaticum)

Description: Cloves, scientifically known as Syzygium aromaticum, are aromatic flower buds from a tree in the Myrtaceae family. Native to the Maluku Islands in Indonesia, cloves are widely used as a spice and in traditional medicine. They are recognized for their strong aroma and flavor, as well as their medicinal properties.

Antibiotic Properties: Cloves possess powerful antibacterial properties primarily due to the presence of eugenol, a potent bioactive compound. Eugenol has been extensively studied for its ability to inhibit the growth of a wide range of bacteria by disrupting their cell walls and membranes. Cloves exhibit broad-spectrum antibacterial activity against pathogens such as Staphylococcus aureus, Escherichia coli, and Helicobacter pylori.

Types of Infections Targeted: Cloves are effective in treating and preventing various internal infections:

- **Oral Infections:** Cloves are highly beneficial for maintaining oral hygiene and preventing infections like toothaches, gingivitis, and periodontitis due to their strong antimicrobial properties.

- **Digestive Infections:** Cloves help combat bacterial infections in the gastrointestinal tract, reducing symptoms of indigestion, gas, and stomach ulcers.
- **Respiratory Infections:** Cloves can aid in treating respiratory infections such as colds, bronchitis, and sinusitis by inhibiting bacterial growth and soothing inflammation.

Dosage Recommendations: For oral use, cloves can be consumed in various forms, including whole, ground, or as clove oil. Generally, 1-2 grams of cloves per day or 2-4 drops of clove oil diluted in a carrier oil are recommended for most therapeutic purposes. It is essential to use clove oil with caution and consult a healthcare provider for personalized dosage recommendations.

Preparation Recipe: *Clove Tea:*

1. **Ingredients:**
   - 4-5 whole cloves
   - 2 cups water
   - Honey or lemon (optional, for taste)

2. **Preparation:**
    - Bring the water to a boil in a saucepan.
    - Add the whole cloves to the boiling water.
    - Reduce the heat and let it simmer for 10-15 minutes.
    - Strain the tea into a cup.
3. **Serving:**
    - Add honey or lemon to taste, if desired.
    - Enjoy the tea warm to benefit from its soothing and antibacterial properties.

Garlic (Allium sativum)

Description: Garlic, scientifically known as Allium sativum, is a bulbous plant in the Allium family, closely related to onions, leeks, and shallots. Originating from Central Asia, garlic has been used for thousands of years for both culinary and medicinal purposes. It is highly regarded for its distinctive flavor and numerous health benefits.

Antibiotic Properties: Garlic is renowned for its potent antibacterial properties, primarily due to the presence of allicin, a sulfur-containing compound. Allicin is formed when garlic is crushed or chopped, and it has been extensively studied for its ability to inhibit the growth of a wide range of bacteria. Garlic's broad-spectrum antibacterial activity is effective against pathogens such as Escherichia coli, Staphylococcus aureus, and Helicobacter pylori. Allicin works by disrupting the cell membranes and metabolic processes of bacteria, preventing their proliferation.

Types of Infections Targeted: Garlic is effective in treating and preventing several internal infections:

- **Respiratory Infections:** Garlic can help combat bacterial infections in the respiratory tract, such as colds, bronchitis, and sinusitis. It also has expectorant properties that aid in relieving congestion.
- **Digestive Infections:** Its antimicrobial properties are beneficial for addressing bacterial infections in the gastrointestinal tract, reducing symptoms of indigestion, bloating, and stomach ulcers.
- **General Immunity:** Garlic enhances immune function, helping the body to fight off infections more effectively and preventing the onset of bacterial diseases.

Dosage Recommendations: For oral use, garlic can be consumed fresh, as garlic powder, or in supplement form. Generally, 1-2 cloves of fresh garlic per day are recommended for most therapeutic purposes. Garlic supplements are often standardized to contain a specific amount of allicin. It is best to consult with a healthcare provider for personalized dosage recommendations.

Preparation Recipe: *Garlic Honey Syrup:*

1. **Ingredients:**
   - 4-5 cloves of fresh garlic
   - 1 cup raw honey
2. **Preparation:**
   - Peel and crush the garlic cloves to activate the allicin.
   - Place the crushed garlic in a small jar.
   - Pour the raw honey over the garlic, ensuring the garlic is fully submerged.
   - Seal the jar and let it sit at room temperature for 3-5 days to allow the flavors to meld and the garlic to infuse the honey.
3. **Serving:**
   - Take 1 teaspoon of the garlic honey syrup daily for its antibacterial benefits.
   - The syrup can be consumed directly, mixed into warm tea, or spread on toast.

This garlic honey syrup recipe provides a natural and effective way to harness the antibacterial benefits of garlic for oral use, promoting respiratory and digestive health and helping to prevent and treat various bacterial infections.

Basil (Ocimum basilicum)

Description: Basil, scientifically known as Ocimum basilicum, is a fragrant herb belonging to the Lamiaceae family. Native to tropical regions from central Africa to Southeast Asia, basil is widely cultivated for its culinary and medicinal uses. It is characterized by its aromatic leaves and small white or purple flowers. Basil has been an integral part of traditional medicine systems, such as Ayurveda and traditional Chinese medicine, for centuries.

Antibiotic Properties: Basil exhibits potent antibacterial properties due to its rich content of essential oils, particularly eugenol, linalool, and estragole. These compounds have been shown to possess strong antibacterial activity, inhibiting the growth of various pathogenic bacteria. Studies have demonstrated that basil essential oil is effective against a wide range of bacteria, including Escherichia coli, Staphylococcus aureus, and Salmonella enteritidis. The antibacterial effects of basil are primarily attributed to its ability to disrupt bacterial cell membranes and inhibit enzyme activity.

Types of Infections Targeted: Basil is effective in treating and preventing several internal infections:

- **Digestive Infections:** Basil helps combat bacterial infections in the gastrointestinal tract, reducing symptoms of indigestion, gas, and bloating. It also supports overall digestive health.
- **Respiratory Infections:** The antibacterial and anti-inflammatory properties of basil make it useful in treating respiratory infections such as colds, bronchitis, and sinusitis.
- **Oral Infections:** Basil can help prevent and treat oral infections, including bad breath, gingivitis, and mouth ulcers.

Dosage Recommendations: For oral use, basil can be consumed fresh, dried, or as an essential oil. Generally, 2-5 grams of fresh basil leaves or 1-2 grams of dried basil leaves per day are recommended. For basil essential oil, 1-2 drops diluted in a carrier oil can be taken internally. It is important to consult with a healthcare provider for personalized dosage recommendations.

Preparation Recipe: *Basil Infused Water:*

1. **Ingredients:**
   - 1 cup fresh basil leaves
   - 1 liter water
   - Lemon slices or honey (optional, for taste)
2. **Preparation:**
   - Wash the fresh basil leaves thoroughly.
   - Slightly crush the basil leaves to release their essential oils.
   - Add the crushed basil leaves to a large pitcher filled with water.
   - Let the basil infuse in the water for at least 2 hours, or overnight in the refrigerator for a stronger flavor.
3. **Serving:**
   - Strain the basil leaves from the water.
   - Add lemon slices or honey to taste, if desired.
   - Drink the basil-infused water throughout the day to benefit from its antibacterial properties.

Cinnamon (Cinnamomum verum)

Description: Cinnamon, scientifically known as Cinnamomum verum, is a spice obtained from the inner bark of trees belonging to the genus Cinnamomum. Native to Sri Lanka and parts of South India, cinnamon has been prized for its aromatic flavor and medicinal properties for thousands of years. It is commonly used in both culinary and medicinal applications, known for its warm, sweet, and slightly spicy taste.

Antibiotic Properties: Cinnamon possesses potent antibacterial properties primarily due to its high content of cinnamaldehyde, a powerful essential oil. Cinnamaldehyde has been shown to inhibit the growth of a wide range of bacteria by disrupting their cell membranes and interfering with their metabolic processes. Studies have demonstrated that cinnamon is effective against various pathogenic bacteria, including Escherichia coli, Staphylococcus aureus, and Salmonella typhi. Additionally, cinnamon's antimicrobial activity extends to antifungal and antiviral properties, making it a versatile natural remedy.

Types of Infections Targeted: Cinnamon is effective in treating and preventing several internal infections:

- **Digestive Infections:** Cinnamon helps combat bacterial infections in the gastrointestinal tract, reducing symptoms of indigestion, gas, and bloating. It also supports overall digestive health and can help prevent foodborne illnesses.
- **Respiratory Infections:** Cinnamon's antibacterial and anti-inflammatory properties make it useful in treating respiratory infections such as colds, bronchitis, and sinusitis.
- **Oral Infections:** Cinnamon can help prevent and treat oral infections, including bad breath, gingivitis, and mouth ulcers, due to its strong antibacterial effects.

Dosage Recommendations: For oral use, cinnamon can be consumed in various forms, including whole sticks, ground powder, or as an essential oil. Generally, 1-2 grams of ground cinnamon per day are recommended for most therapeutic purposes. For cinnamon essential oil, 1-2 drops diluted in a carrier oil can be taken internally. It is important to consult with a healthcare provider for personalized dosage recommendations.

Preparation Recipe: *Cinnamon Honey Elixir:*

1. **Ingredients:**
   - 1 teaspoon ground cinnamon
   - 1 tablespoon raw honey
   - 1 cup warm water or herbal tea
2. **Preparation:**
   - Mix the ground cinnamon and raw honey together in a small bowl to form a paste.
   - Add the cinnamon-honey paste to a cup of warm water or herbal tea.
   - Stir well to dissolve the mixture.
3. **Serving:**
   - Drink the cinnamon honey elixir once or twice daily to benefit from its antibacterial properties.
   - This elixir can be consumed on an empty stomach or before meals to enhance digestion and boost immunity.

Sage (Salvia officinalis)

Description: Sage, scientifically known as Salvia officinalis, is a perennial herb in the mint family, Lamiaceae. Native to the Mediterranean region, sage has been used for centuries in both culinary and medicinal contexts. The herb is characterized by its grayish-green leaves and woody stems, as well as its strong, earthy aroma and slightly peppery flavor.

Antibiotic Properties: Sage is renowned for its potent antibacterial properties, which are primarily attributed to its essential oils, such as thujone, camphor, and cineole. These compounds exhibit strong antibacterial activity by disrupting the cell membranes of bacteria and inhibiting their metabolic functions. Research has shown that sage is effective against a wide range of pathogenic bacteria, including Escherichia coli, Staphylococcus aureus, and Salmonella typhi. Additionally, sage has antifungal and antiviral properties, enhancing its overall antimicrobial efficacy.

Types of Infections Targeted: Sage is effective in treating and preventing several internal infections:

- **Respiratory Infections:** Sage is beneficial for treating respiratory infections such as colds, bronchitis, and sore throats. Its antibacterial properties help eliminate pathogens, while its anti-inflammatory effects soothe the respiratory tract.
- **Digestive Infections:** Sage aids in combating bacterial infections in the gastrointestinal tract, reducing symptoms of indigestion, bloating, and diarrhea.
- **Oral Infections:** Sage is highly effective in maintaining oral hygiene and preventing infections such as gingivitis, periodontitis, and mouth ulcers.

Dosage Recommendations: For oral use, sage can be consumed fresh, dried, or as an essential oil. Generally, 1-2 grams of dried sage leaves per day are recommended, or 2-4 drops of sage essential oil diluted in a carrier oil. Sage tea is a common method of consumption. It is important to consult with a healthcare provider for personalized dosage recommendations, especially when using sage essential oil.

Preparation Recipe: *Sage Tea:*

1. **Ingredients:**
   - 1-2 teaspoons dried sage leaves (or 5-6 fresh sage leaves)
   - 1 cup boiling water
   - Honey or lemon (optional, for taste)
2. **Preparation:**
   - Place the dried sage leaves or fresh sage leaves in a tea infuser or teapot.
   - Pour the boiling water over the sage.
   - Cover and let it steep for 5-10 minutes.
   - Strain the tea into a cup.
3. **Serving:**
   - Add honey or lemon to taste, if desired.
   - Enjoy the tea warm to benefit from its soothing and antibacterial properties.

Grapefruit Seed Extract (Citrus paradisi)

Description: Grapefruit Seed Extract (GSE), derived from the seeds, pulp, and white membranes of grapefruit (Citrus paradisi), is a potent natural remedy with a range of medicinal applications. Originating from Southeast Asia, grapefruit is now widely grown in subtropical and tropical regions around the world. GSE is known for its strong antimicrobial properties and is commonly used in dietary supplements, personal care products, and cleaning agents.

Antibiotic Properties: GSE is renowned for its broad-spectrum antibacterial properties, primarily due to its high content of bioflavonoids and polyphenolic compounds such as naringenin, hesperidin, and quercetin. These compounds work by disrupting the cell membranes of bacteria and interfering with their enzyme activity, leading to the inhibition of bacterial growth. Studies have demonstrated that GSE is effective against a wide range of pathogenic bacteria, including Escherichia coli, Staphylococcus aureus, and Salmonella spp. Additionally, GSE exhibits antifungal and antiviral properties, enhancing its overall antimicrobial efficacy.

Types of Infections Targeted: GSE is effective in treating and preventing several internal infections:

- **Digestive Infections:** GSE helps combat bacterial infections in the gastrointestinal tract, reducing symptoms of indigestion, bloating, and diarrhea. It also supports overall digestive health by balancing gut flora.
- **Respiratory Infections:** The antibacterial and antiviral properties of GSE make it useful in treating respiratory infections such as colds, bronchitis, and sinusitis.
- **Oral Infections:** GSE is beneficial for maintaining oral hygiene and preventing infections such as gingivitis, periodontitis, and bad breath.

Dosage Recommendations: For oral use, GSE can be consumed as a liquid extract or in capsule form. Generally, 10-15 drops of GSE diluted in a glass of water or juice, taken 1-3 times daily, is recommended for most therapeutic purposes. GSE capsules are often standardized to contain a specific amount of the active compounds. It is important to consult with a healthcare provider for personalized dosage recommendations.

Preparation Recipe: *Grapefruit Seed Extract Gargle:*

1. **Ingredients:**
   - 10-15 drops of GSE
   - 1 cup warm water
   - Honey or salt (optional, for taste and additional soothing properties)
2. **Preparation:**
   - Add the GSE drops to the warm water.
   - Stir well to ensure the extract is evenly distributed.
3. **Serving:**
   - Gargle with the solution for 30 seconds to 1 minute, then spit it out.
   - Repeat this process 2-3 times daily to help treat and prevent oral and respiratory infections.
   - For enhanced soothing, add a teaspoon of honey or salt to the solution.

Licorice (Glycyrrhiza glabra)

Description: Licorice, scientifically known as Glycyrrhiza glabra, is a perennial herb native to the Mediterranean and parts of Asia. It has been used for thousands of years in traditional medicine systems, such as Ayurveda and traditional Chinese medicine, for its sweet flavor and numerous health benefits. The root of the licorice plant is most commonly used for medicinal purposes.

Antibiotic Properties: Licorice exhibits significant antibacterial properties primarily due to its active compound, glycyrrhizin. Glycyrrhizin and other bioactive compounds in licorice, such as flavonoids, have been shown to inhibit the growth of various bacteria by disrupting their cell walls and interfering with their metabolic processes. Research indicates that licorice is effective against a broad range of bacteria, including Staphylococcus aureus, Escherichia coli, and Helicobacter pylori. Additionally, licorice possesses antiviral and antifungal properties, making it a versatile antimicrobial agent.

Types of Infections Targeted: Licorice is effective in treating and preventing several internal infections:

- **Respiratory Infections:** Licorice is beneficial for treating respiratory infections such as sore throats, bronchitis, and colds due to its antibacterial and anti-inflammatory properties. It helps soothe the respiratory tract and reduce symptoms.
- **Digestive Infections:** Licorice can help combat bacterial infections in the gastrointestinal tract, reducing symptoms of indigestion, gastritis, and ulcers. It also promotes overall digestive health.
- **Oral Infections:** Licorice is useful in preventing and treating oral infections, including gingivitis, periodontitis, and mouth ulcers, due to its strong antibacterial effects.

Dosage Recommendations: For oral use, licorice can be consumed as a dried root, powder, or extract. Generally, 1-2 grams of dried licorice root or 300-600 mg of licorice extract per day are recommended for most therapeutic purposes. It is important to consult with a healthcare provider for personalized dosage recommendations, especially for long-term use, as excessive consumption of licorice can lead to adverse effects.

Preparation Recipe: *Licorice Root Tea:*

1. **Ingredients:**
    - 1-2 teaspoons dried licorice root
    - 1 cup boiling water
    - Honey or lemon (optional, for taste)
2. **Preparation:**
    - Place the dried licorice root in a tea infuser or teapot.
    - Pour the boiling water over the licorice root.
    - Cover and let it steep for 10-15 minutes.
    - Strain the tea into a cup.
3. **Serving:**
    - Add honey or lemon to taste, if desired.
    - Drink the tea warm to benefit from its soothing and antibacterial properties.
    - Enjoy 1-2 cups daily to help prevent and treat various bacterial infections.

Cranberry (Vaccinium macrocarpon)

Description: Cranberry, scientifically known as Vaccinium macrocarpon, is a small, evergreen shrub native to North America. The berries are well known for their tart flavor and are widely used in both culinary and medicinal applications. Cranberries have been valued for their health benefits for centuries, particularly in preventing and treating urinary tract infections (UTIs).

Antibiotic Properties: Cranberries possess significant antibacterial properties primarily due to their high content of proanthocyanidins (PACs) and other phenolic compounds. These compounds inhibit the adhesion of bacteria, particularly Escherichia coli, to the walls of the urinary tract, preventing infection. Cranberries also contain organic acids like hippuric acid, which have a bacteriostatic effect, further contributing to their antimicrobial activity. While cranberries are most famous for their use in urinary health, their antibacterial properties extend to other areas as well.

Types of Infections Targeted: Cranberries are effective in treating and preventing several internal infections:

- **Urinary Tract Infections (UTIs):** Cranberries are particularly effective in preventing and treating UTIs by preventing the adhesion of E. coli bacteria to the urinary tract lining.
- **Digestive Infections:** The antibacterial properties of cranberries can help maintain gut health and prevent digestive infections, reducing symptoms like indigestion and bloating.
- **Oral Infections:** Cranberries can also contribute to oral health by inhibiting the growth of bacteria that cause gum disease and cavities.

Dosage Recommendations: For oral use, cranberries can be consumed fresh, as juice, or in supplement form. Generally, 8-16 ounces of unsweetened cranberry juice or 500 mg of cranberry extract twice daily are recommended for most therapeutic purposes. It is important to consult with a healthcare provider for personalized dosage recommendations.

Preparation Recipe: *Cranberry Juice:*

1. **Ingredients:**
    - 1 cup fresh or frozen cranberries
    - 4 cups water

- o Honey or stevia (optional, for taste)

2. **Preparation:**
   - o Rinse the cranberries thoroughly.
   - o In a large pot, combine the cranberries and water.
   - o Bring to a boil, then reduce heat and simmer for about 15 minutes until the cranberries burst.
   - o Remove from heat and let the mixture cool slightly.
   - o Strain the juice through a fine mesh strainer or cheesecloth into a pitcher, pressing the cranberries to extract all the juice.
   - o Add honey or stevia to taste, if desired.

3. **Serving:**
   - o Refrigerate the juice and serve chilled.
   - o Drink 8-16 ounces of cranberry juice daily to benefit from its antibacterial properties and prevent urinary tract infections.

Bergamot (Citrus bergamia)

Description: Bergamot, scientifically known as Citrus bergamia, is a citrus fruit native to the Mediterranean region. It is a hybrid of bitter orange and lemon, renowned for its distinctive fragrance and essential oil, which is extracted from the fruit's rind. Bergamot essential oil is widely used in aromatherapy, perfumery, and traditional medicine for its numerous health benefits.

Antibiotic Properties: Bergamot possesses significant antibacterial properties due to its high content of compounds such as linalool, limonene, and linalyl acetate. These compounds have been shown to inhibit the growth of various pathogenic bacteria by disrupting their cell membranes and interfering with their metabolic processes. Studies indicate that bergamot essential oil is effective against a wide range of bacteria, including Escherichia coli, Staphylococcus aureus, and Listeria monocytogenes. Additionally, bergamot exhibits antifungal and antiviral properties, making it a versatile antimicrobial agent.

Types of Infections Targeted: Bergamot is effective in treating and preventing several internal infections:

- **Respiratory Infections:** Bergamot essential oil is beneficial for treating respiratory infections such as colds, bronchitis, and sinusitis. Its antibacterial and anti-inflammatory properties help eliminate pathogens and soothe the respiratory tract.
- **Digestive Infections:** Bergamot aids in combating bacterial infections in the gastrointestinal tract, reducing symptoms of indigestion, bloating, and stomach ulcers.
- **Oral Infections:** Bergamot can help maintain oral hygiene and prevent infections such as gingivitis, periodontitis, and mouth ulcers due to its strong antibacterial effects.

Dosage Recommendations: For oral use, bergamot essential oil should be used with caution and only in diluted form. Generally, 1-2 drops of bergamot essential oil diluted in a carrier oil or water, taken 1-2 times daily, is recommended for most therapeutic purposes. It is crucial to consult with a healthcare provider for personalized dosage recommendations and to ensure safe usage, as bergamot essential oil can be phototoxic and should not be used in large quantities.

Preparation Recipe: *Bergamot Honey Elixir:*

1. **Ingredients:**
   - 1-2 drops of bergamot essential oil
   - 1 tablespoon raw honey
   - 1 cup warm water or herbal tea
2. **Preparation:**
   - Add the bergamot essential oil to the raw honey and mix well to combine.
   - Stir the honey mixture into a cup of warm water or herbal tea until fully dissolved.
3. **Serving:**
   - Drink the bergamot honey elixir once or twice daily to benefit from its antibacterial properties.
   - This elixir can be consumed on an empty stomach or before meals to enhance digestion and boost immunity.

Lemongrass (Cymbopogon citratus)

Description: Lemongrass, scientifically known as Cymbopogon citratus, is a tall, perennial grass native to tropical and subtropical regions of Asia. It is widely used in culinary, medicinal, and aromatherapy applications. The plant is known for its strong citrus aroma and flavor, which comes from its essential oils, particularly citral and limonene.

Antibiotic Properties: Lemongrass possesses significant antibacterial properties due to its high content of essential oils such as citral, limonene, and geraniol. These compounds exhibit strong antibacterial activity by disrupting the cell membranes of bacteria and interfering with their metabolic processes. Research has shown that lemongrass essential oil is effective against a broad spectrum of bacteria, including Escherichia coli, Staphylococcus aureus, and Salmonella typhi. Additionally, lemongrass has antifungal and antiviral properties, enhancing its overall antimicrobial efficacy.

Types of Infections Targeted: Lemongrass is effective in treating and preventing several internal infections:

- **Digestive Infections:** Lemongrass helps combat bacterial infections in the gastrointestinal tract, reducing symptoms of indigestion, bloating, and diarrhea. It also supports overall digestive health by promoting healthy gut flora.
- **Respiratory Infections:** The antibacterial and antiviral properties of lemongrass make it useful in treating respiratory infections such as colds, bronchitis, and sinusitis.
- **Oral Infections:** Lemongrass can help prevent and treat oral infections, including bad breath, gingivitis, and mouth ulcers, due to its strong antibacterial effects.

Dosage Recommendations: For oral use, lemongrass can be consumed as fresh or dried leaves, tea, or essential oil. Generally, 1-2 grams of dried lemongrass leaves or 1-2 drops of lemongrass essential oil diluted in a carrier oil per day are recommended for most therapeutic purposes. It is important to consult with a healthcare provider for personalized dosage recommendations, especially when using lemongrass essential oil.

Preparation Recipe: *Lemongrass Tea:*

1. **Ingredients:**
    - 1-2 teaspoons dried lemongrass leaves (or 1-2 fresh lemongrass stalks, chopped)
    - 1 cup boiling water
    - Honey or lemon (optional, for taste)
2. **Preparation:**
    - Place the dried lemongrass leaves or chopped fresh lemongrass in a tea infuser or teapot.
    - Pour the boiling water over the lemongrass.
    - Cover and let it steep for 5-10 minutes.
    - Strain the tea into a cup.
3. **Serving:**
    - Add honey or lemon to taste, if desired.
    - Drink the tea warm to benefit from its soothing and antibacterial properties.
    - Enjoy 1-2 cups daily to help prevent and treat various bacterial infections.

Peppermint (Mentha piperita)

Description: Peppermint, scientifically known as Mentha piperita, is a hybrid mint, a cross between watermint and spearmint. Native to Europe and the Middle East, it is now widely cultivated across the globe. Peppermint is characterized by its aromatic leaves and refreshing, cool flavor, which comes from its high menthol content. The leaves and essential oil of peppermint are commonly used for their medicinal properties.

Antibiotic Properties: Peppermint exhibits significant antibacterial properties primarily due to its high menthol and menthone content. These compounds are known to disrupt bacterial cell membranes and inhibit their growth. Studies have shown that peppermint oil is effective against a wide range of bacteria, including Escherichia coli, Staphylococcus aureus, and Salmonella enterica. Additionally, peppermint possesses antifungal and antiviral properties, enhancing its overall antimicrobial activity.

Types of Infections Targeted: Peppermint is effective in treating and preventing several internal infections:

- **Digestive Infections:** Peppermint helps combat bacterial infections in the gastrointestinal tract, alleviating symptoms of indigestion, bloating, and irritable bowel syndrome (IBS). It also promotes overall digestive health.
- **Respiratory Infections:** Peppermint's antibacterial and antiviral properties make it useful in treating respiratory infections such as colds, bronchitis, and sinusitis. It helps clear nasal congestion and soothe the respiratory tract.
- **Oral Infections:** Peppermint can help maintain oral hygiene and prevent infections such as gingivitis, periodontitis, and bad breath due to its strong antibacterial effects.

Dosage Recommendations: For oral use, peppermint can be consumed as fresh or dried leaves, tea, or essential oil. Generally, 1-2 grams of dried peppermint leaves or 1-2 drops of peppermint essential oil diluted in a carrier oil or water per day are recommended for most therapeutic purposes. It is important to consult with a healthcare provider for personalized dosage recommendations.

Preparation Recipe: *Peppermint Tea:*

1. **Ingredients:**
   - 1-2 teaspoons dried peppermint leaves (or a few fresh peppermint leaves)
   - 1 cup boiling water
   - Honey or lemon (optional, for taste)
2. **Preparation:**
   - Place the dried peppermint leaves or fresh peppermint leaves in a tea infuser or teapot.
   - Pour the boiling water over the peppermint.
   - Cover and let it steep for 5-10 minutes.
   - Strain the tea into a cup.
3. **Serving:**
   - Add honey or lemon to taste, if desired.
   - Drink the tea warm to benefit from its soothing and antibacterial properties.
   - Enjoy 1-2 cups daily to help prevent and treat various bacterial infections.

Angelica (Angelica archangelica)

Description: Angelica, scientifically known as Angelica archangelica, is a biennial plant native to northern Europe and Asia. It has been used for centuries in traditional medicine for its wide range of therapeutic properties. The plant features large, umbrella-like clusters of greenish-white flowers and aromatic, hollow stems. Both the root and aerial parts of the plant are used for medicinal purposes.

Antibiotic Properties: Angelica possesses significant antibacterial properties due to its high content of essential oils and bioactive compounds such as coumarins, flavonoids, and polyacetylenes. These compounds have been shown to inhibit the growth of various pathogenic bacteria by disrupting their cell membranes and interfering with their metabolic processes. Research indicates that angelica is effective against a broad spectrum of bacteria, including Escherichia coli, Staphylococcus aureus, and Bacillus subtilis. Additionally, angelica has antifungal and antiviral properties, enhancing its overall antimicrobial efficacy.

Types of Infections Targeted: Angelica is effective in treating and preventing several internal infections:

- **Respiratory Infections:** Angelica is beneficial for treating respiratory infections such as colds, bronchitis, and sinusitis. Its antibacterial and anti-inflammatory properties help eliminate pathogens and soothe the respiratory tract.
- **Digestive Infections:** Angelica aids in combating bacterial infections in the gastrointestinal tract, reducing symptoms of indigestion, bloating, and flatulence. It also supports overall digestive health by promoting healthy gut flora.
- **Oral Infections:** Angelica can help maintain oral hygiene and prevent infections such as gingivitis, periodontitis, and mouth ulcers due to its strong antibacterial effects.

Dosage Recommendations: For oral use, angelica can be consumed as a dried root, tea, or tincture. Generally, 1-2 grams of dried angelica root or 1-2 ml of angelica tincture taken 2-3 times daily are recommended for most therapeutic purposes. It is important to consult with a healthcare provider for personalized dosage recommendations, especially for long-term use.

Preparation Recipe: *Angelica Root Tea:*

1. **Ingredients:**
   - 1-2 teaspoons dried angelica root
   - 1 cup boiling water
   - Honey or lemon (optional, for taste)
2. **Preparation:**
   - Place the dried angelica root in a tea infuser or teapot.
   - Pour the boiling water over the angelica root.
   - Cover and let it steep for 10-15 minutes.
   - Strain the tea into a cup.
3. **Serving:**
   - Add honey or lemon to taste, if desired.
   - Drink the tea warm to benefit from its soothing and antibacterial properties.
   - Enjoy 1-2 cups daily to help prevent and treat various bacterial infections.

Cat's Claw (Uncaria tomentosa)

Description: Cat's Claw, scientifically known as Uncaria tomentosa, is a woody vine native to the Amazon rainforest and other tropical areas of South and Central America. It gets its name from the thorns on the plant, which resemble a cat's claw. Traditionally used by indigenous peoples for its medicinal properties, Cat's Claw has garnered attention for its immune-boosting and anti-inflammatory effects. Both the bark and root of the plant are utilized in herbal medicine.

Antibiotic Properties: Cat's Claw exhibits notable antibacterial properties primarily due to its rich content of oxindole alkaloids, quinovic acid glycosides, and polyphenols. These compounds have demonstrated the ability to inhibit the growth of various pathogenic bacteria by disrupting their cell walls and metabolic processes. Studies have shown that Cat's Claw is effective against bacteria such as Escherichia coli, Staphylococcus aureus, and Helicobacter pylori. Additionally, Cat's Claw has antifungal and antiviral properties, further enhancing its antimicrobial profile.

Types of Infections Targeted: Cat's Claw is effective in treating and preventing several internal infections:

- **Digestive Infections:** Cat's Claw helps combat bacterial infections in the gastrointestinal tract, alleviating symptoms of stomach ulcers, gastritis, and inflammatory bowel diseases.
- **Respiratory Infections:** Its antibacterial and antiviral properties make Cat's Claw useful in treating respiratory infections such as colds, bronchitis, and sinusitis.
- **Urinary Tract Infections (UTIs):** Cat's Claw can assist in preventing and treating UTIs by inhibiting the adhesion of bacteria to the urinary tract lining.

Dosage Recommendations: For oral use, Cat's Claw can be consumed as a tea, capsule, or tincture. Generally, 250-350 mg of Cat's Claw extract taken 2-3 times daily or 1-2 ml of Cat's Claw tincture taken 1-2 times daily are recommended for most therapeutic purposes. It is crucial to consult with a healthcare provider for personalized dosage recommendations, especially if using Cat's Claw for extended periods.

Preparation Recipe: *Cat's Claw Tea:*

1. **Ingredients:**
    - 1-2 teaspoons dried Cat's Claw bark or root
    - 1 cup boiling water
    - Honey or lemon (optional, for taste)
2. **Preparation:**
    - Place the dried Cat's Claw bark or root in a tea infuser or teapot.
    - Pour the boiling water over the Cat's Claw.
    - Cover and let it steep for 15-20 minutes.
    - Strain the tea into a cup.
3. **Serving:**
    - Add honey or lemon to taste, if desired.
    - Drink the tea warm to benefit from its soothing and antibacterial properties.
    - Enjoy 1-2 cups daily to help prevent and treat various bacterial infections.

Elderberry (Sambucus nigra)

Description: Elderberry, scientifically known as Sambucus nigra, is a deciduous shrub or small tree native to Europe. It produces clusters of small, dark purple berries and white or cream-colored flowers. The berries and flowers of the elderberry plant have been used for centuries in traditional medicine due to their numerous health benefits. Elderberry is renowned for its immune-boosting properties and is commonly used to treat colds and flu.

Antibiotic Properties: Elderberry exhibits notable antibacterial properties attributed to its high content of flavonoids, anthocyanins, and phenolic acids. These compounds have demonstrated the ability to inhibit the growth of various pathogenic bacteria by disrupting their cell walls and metabolic processes. Studies have shown that elderberry extracts are effective against bacteria such as Streptococcus pyogenes, Branhamella catarrhalis, and Haemophilus influenzae. Additionally, elderberry has strong antiviral properties, which further enhance its antimicrobial efficacy.

Types of Infections Targeted: Elderberry is effective in treating and preventing several internal infections:

- **Respiratory Infections:** Elderberry is particularly beneficial for treating respiratory infections such as colds, flu, bronchitis, and sinusitis. Its antibacterial and antiviral properties help eliminate pathogens and reduce the duration and severity of symptoms.
- **Digestive Infections:** Elderberry can help combat bacterial infections in the gastrointestinal tract, alleviating symptoms of indigestion and promoting overall digestive health.
- **Urinary Tract Infections (UTIs):** Elderberry's antimicrobial properties make it useful in preventing and treating UTIs by inhibiting the growth of bacteria in the urinary tract.

Dosage Recommendations: For oral use, elderberry can be consumed as fresh or dried berries, syrup, or extract. Generally, 1-2 tablespoons of elderberry syrup taken 2-3 times daily or 250-500 mg of elderberry extract taken 1-2 times daily are recommended for most therapeutic purposes. It is essential to consult with a healthcare provider for personalized dosage recommendations.

Preparation Recipe: *Elderberry Syrup:*

1. **Ingredients:**
   - 1 cup dried elderberries (or 2 cups fresh elderberries)
   - 4 cups water
   - 1 cup raw honey
   - 1 cinnamon stick (optional)
   - 1-2 cloves (optional)
   - 1 piece of fresh ginger, sliced (optional)
2. **Preparation:**
   - In a medium saucepan, combine the elderberries, water, and optional ingredients (cinnamon stick, cloves, and ginger).
   - Bring the mixture to a boil, then reduce the heat and let it simmer for 45 minutes to an hour, until the liquid has reduced by about half.
   - Remove the saucepan from heat and let it cool slightly.
   - Mash the elderberries using a spoon or potato masher, then strain the mixture through a fine

mesh strainer or cheesecloth into
a bowl.

- Discard the solids and allow the
  liquid to cool to lukewarm
  temperature.
- Stir in the raw honey until well
  combined.

3. **Serving:**

- Pour the elderberry syrup into a
  clean glass jar or bottle and store
  it in the refrigerator.
- Take 1-2 tablespoons of the syrup
  daily to boost immunity and help
  prevent and treat bacterial
  infections.
- The syrup can be taken on its own
  or added to water, tea, or
  smoothies.

Horseradish (Armoracia rusticana)

Description: Horseradish, scientifically known as Armoracia rusticana, is a perennial plant belonging to the Brassicaceae family, which also includes mustard, wasabi, and cabbage. Native to southeastern Europe and western Asia, horseradish is now cultivated worldwide. The plant is known for its large, white, tapered root, which has a pungent and spicy flavor. The root is typically grated or ground and used as a condiment, but it also has a long history of medicinal use.

Antibiotic Properties: Horseradish has potent antibacterial properties due to its high content of glucosinolates and their breakdown products, such as allyl isothiocyanate. These compounds have been shown to inhibit the growth of a variety of bacteria by disrupting their cell walls and metabolic processes. Studies have demonstrated that horseradish is effective against bacteria such as Escherichia coli, Staphylococcus aureus, and Pseudomonas aeruginosa. Additionally, horseradish has antifungal and antiviral properties, enhancing its overall antimicrobial efficacy.

Types of Infections Targeted: Horseradish is effective in treating and preventing several internal infections:

- **Respiratory Infections:** Horseradish is particularly beneficial for treating respiratory infections such as colds, sinusitis, and bronchitis. Its antibacterial and mucolytic properties help clear nasal congestion, reduce mucus production, and eliminate pathogens.
- **Urinary Tract Infections (UTIs):** Horseradish can assist in preventing and treating UTIs by inhibiting the growth of bacteria in the urinary tract and promoting the elimination of toxins through increased urine flow.
- **Digestive Infections:** Horseradish aids in combating bacterial infections in the gastrointestinal tract, reducing symptoms of indigestion and promoting overall digestive health.

Dosage Recommendations: For oral use, horseradish can be consumed as fresh root, tincture, or prepared condiment. Generally, 1-2 teaspoons of freshly grated horseradish root taken 2-3 times daily or 1-2 ml of horseradish tincture taken 1-2 times daily are recommended for most therapeutic purposes. It is important to consult with a healthcare provider for personalized dosage recommendations, especially for long-term use.

Preparation Recipe: *Horseradish Infusion:*

1. **Ingredients:**
   - 2-3 teaspoons freshly grated horseradish root
   - 1 cup hot (not boiling) water
   - Honey or lemon (optional, for taste)
2. **Preparation:**
   - Place the freshly grated horseradish root in a cup or mug.
   - Pour the hot water over the horseradish.
   - Cover and let it steep for 10-15 minutes.
   - Strain the infusion into another cup or mug.
3. **Serving:**
   - Add honey or lemon to taste, if desired.
   - Drink the infusion warm to benefit from its soothing and antibacterial properties.

- ○ Enjoy 1-2 cups daily to help
  prevent and treat various
  bacterial infections.

Juniper (Juniperus communis)

Description: Juniper, scientifically known as Juniperus communis, is an evergreen shrub or small tree that belongs to the cypress family (Cupressaceae). It is widely distributed across the Northern Hemisphere, particularly in Europe, Asia, and North America. Juniper is recognized by its needle-like leaves and small, fleshy, berry-like cones known as juniper berries. These berries have been used for centuries in traditional medicine and as a spice in culinary applications.

Antibiotic Properties: Juniper berries exhibit strong antibacterial properties due to their high content of essential oils, particularly terpinen-4-ol, alpha-pinene, and beta-myrcene. These compounds have been shown to inhibit the growth of a variety of pathogenic bacteria by disrupting their cell membranes and metabolic processes. Studies have demonstrated that juniper berry extracts are effective against bacteria such as Escherichia coli, Staphylococcus aureus, and Bacillus subtilis. Additionally, juniper has antifungal and antiviral properties, enhancing its overall antimicrobial profile.

Types of Infections Targeted: Juniper is effective in treating and preventing several internal infections:

- **Urinary Tract Infections (UTIs):** Juniper berries are particularly beneficial for treating UTIs. Their diuretic and antibacterial properties help flush out bacteria from the urinary tract and reduce inflammation.
- **Respiratory Infections:** Juniper can assist in alleviating symptoms of respiratory infections such as colds, bronchitis, and sinusitis. Its antibacterial and anti-inflammatory properties help clear congestion and eliminate pathogens.
- **Digestive Infections:** Juniper berries aid in combating bacterial infections in the gastrointestinal tract, reducing symptoms of indigestion, bloating, and gas.

Dosage Recommendations: For oral use, juniper berries can be consumed as dried berries, tea, or tincture. Generally, 1-2 grams of dried juniper berries or 1-2 ml of juniper tincture taken 1-2 times daily are recommended for most therapeutic purposes. It is crucial to consult with a healthcare provider for personalized dosage recommendations, especially for long-term use and for those with kidney conditions, as juniper is a strong diuretic.

Preparation Recipe: *Juniper Berry Tea:*

1. **Ingredients:**
   - 1 teaspoon dried juniper berries
   - 1 cup boiling water
   - Honey or lemon (optional, for taste)
2. **Preparation:**
   - Crush the dried juniper berries slightly to release their essential oils.
   - Place the crushed juniper berries in a tea infuser or teapot.
   - Pour the boiling water over the juniper berries.
   - Cover and let it steep for 10-15 minutes.
   - Strain the tea into a cup.
3. **Serving:**
   - Add honey or lemon to taste, if desired.
   - Drink the tea warm to benefit from its soothing and antibacterial properties.

o   Enjoy 1-2 cups daily to help prevent and treat various bacterial infections.

This juniper berry tea recipe provides a natural and effective way to harness the antibacterial benefits of juniper for oral use, promoting urinary, respiratory, and digestive health and helping to prevent and treat various bacterial infections.

Nasturtium (Tropaeolum majus)

Description: Nasturtium, scientifically known as Tropaeolum majus, is a flowering plant native to South America. It is prized for its vibrant, trumpet-shaped flowers and rounded, shield-like leaves. Nasturtium is widely grown as an ornamental plant, but its leaves, flowers, and seeds are also edible and have been used in traditional medicine for their numerous health benefits.

Antibiotic Properties: Nasturtium exhibits significant antibacterial properties due to its high content of mustard oil glycosides, such as benzyl isothiocyanate, and other bioactive compounds. These compounds have demonstrated the ability to inhibit the growth of various pathogenic bacteria by disrupting their cell walls and metabolic processes. Studies have shown that nasturtium is effective against bacteria such as Escherichia coli, Staphylococcus aureus, and Pseudomonas aeruginosa. Additionally, nasturtium has antifungal and antiviral properties, further enhancing its antimicrobial profile.

Types of Infections Targeted: Nasturtium is effective in treating and preventing several internal infections:

- **Respiratory Infections:** Nasturtium is beneficial for treating respiratory infections such as colds, bronchitis, and sinusitis. Its antibacterial and anti-inflammatory properties help eliminate pathogens and reduce symptoms.
- **Urinary Tract Infections (UTIs):** Nasturtium can assist in preventing and treating UTIs by inhibiting the growth of bacteria in the urinary tract and promoting the elimination of toxins through increased urine flow.
- **Digestive Infections:** Nasturtium aids in combating bacterial infections in the gastrointestinal tract, reducing symptoms of indigestion and promoting overall digestive health.

Dosage Recommendations: For oral use, nasturtium can be consumed as fresh leaves and flowers, tea, or tincture. Generally, 1-2 grams of dried nasturtium or 1-2 ml of nasturtium tincture taken 1-2 times daily are recommended for most therapeutic purposes. It is essential to consult with a healthcare provider for personalized dosage recommendations.

Preparation Recipe: *Nasturtium Tea:*

1. **Ingredients:**
   - 1-2 teaspoons dried nasturtium leaves and flowers
   - 1 cup boiling water
   - Honey or lemon (optional, for taste)
2. **Preparation:**
   - Place the dried nasturtium leaves and flowers in a tea infuser or teapot.
   - Pour the boiling water over the nasturtium.
   - Cover and let it steep for 10-15 minutes.
   - Strain the tea into a cup.
3. **Serving:**
   - Add honey or lemon to taste, if desired.
   - Drink the tea warm to benefit from its soothing and antibacterial properties.
   - Enjoy 1-2 cups daily to help prevent and treat various bacterial infections.

Pau d'Arco (Tabebuia impetiginosa)

Description: Pau d'Arco, scientifically known as Tabebuia impetiginosa, is a tropical tree native to the Amazon rainforest and other tropical regions of South and Central America. The tree is known for its hard, dense wood and beautiful pink-to-purple flowers. The inner bark of Pau d'Arco has been used for centuries by indigenous peoples for its medicinal properties. It is traditionally consumed as a tea or tincture and is renowned for its wide range of health benefits.

Antibiotic Properties: Pau d'Arco possesses potent antibacterial properties primarily due to its high content of naphthoquinones, particularly lapachol and beta-lapachone. These compounds have demonstrated the ability to inhibit the growth of a variety of pathogenic bacteria by disrupting their cell membranes and metabolic processes. Studies have shown that Pau d'Arco is effective against bacteria such as Staphylococcus aureus, Escherichia coli, and Helicobacter pylori. Additionally, Pau d'Arco has antifungal and antiviral properties, further enhancing its antimicrobial profile.

Types of Infections Targeted: Pau d'Arco is effective in treating and preventing several internal infections:

- **Respiratory Infections:** Pau d'Arco can be used to treat respiratory infections such as colds, bronchitis, and sinusitis. Its antibacterial and antiviral properties help eliminate pathogens and reduce symptoms.
- **Digestive Infections:** Pau d'Arco aids in combating bacterial infections in the gastrointestinal tract, reducing symptoms of indigestion and promoting overall digestive health.
- **Urinary Tract Infections (UTIs):** Pau d'Arco's antimicrobial properties make it useful in preventing and treating UTIs by inhibiting the growth of bacteria in the urinary tract.

Dosage Recommendations: For oral use, Pau d'Arco can be consumed as a tea, capsule, or tincture. Generally, 1-2 grams of Pau d'Arco bark or 1-2 ml of Pau d'Arco tincture taken 1-2 times daily are recommended for most therapeutic purposes. It is essential to consult with a healthcare provider for personalized dosage recommendations, especially for long-term use.

Preparation Recipe: *Pau d'Arco Tea:*

1. **Ingredients:**
   - 1-2 teaspoons dried Pau d'Arco bark
   - 1 cup boiling water
   - Honey or lemon (optional, for taste)
2. **Preparation:**
   - Place the dried Pau d'Arco bark in a tea infuser or teapot.
   - Pour the boiling water over the Pau d'Arco.
   - Cover and let it steep for 15-20 minutes.
   - Strain the tea into a cup.
3. **Serving:**
   - Add honey or lemon to taste, if desired.
   - Drink the tea warm to benefit from its soothing and antibacterial properties.
   - Enjoy 1-2 cups daily to help prevent and treat various bacterial infections.

Propolis

Description: Propolis is a resinous mixture produced by honey bees by combining their saliva and beeswax with exudate gathered from tree buds, sap flows, or other botanical sources. The bees use propolis to seal small gaps in the hive, creating a sterile environment and protecting it from external threats. Propolis has been used for centuries in traditional medicine for its impressive range of health benefits, particularly its antimicrobial properties.

Antibiotic Properties: Propolis exhibits significant antibacterial properties due to its rich composition of flavonoids, phenolic acids, and essential oils. These compounds have been shown to inhibit the growth of various pathogenic bacteria by disrupting their cell walls and metabolic processes. Studies have demonstrated that propolis is effective against bacteria such as Staphylococcus aureus, Escherichia coli, and Helicobacter pylori. Additionally, propolis has antifungal, antiviral, and anti-inflammatory properties, further enhancing its antimicrobial efficacy.

Types of Infections Targeted: Propolis is effective in treating and preventing several internal infections:

- **Respiratory Infections:** Propolis is beneficial for treating respiratory infections such as colds, bronchitis, and sinusitis. Its antibacterial and antiviral properties help eliminate pathogens and reduce symptoms.
- **Digestive Infections:** Propolis can help combat bacterial infections in the gastrointestinal tract, reducing symptoms of indigestion and promoting overall digestive health.
- **Oral Infections:** Propolis is particularly useful in treating oral infections such as gingivitis, periodontitis, and canker sores. Its antibacterial properties help reduce inflammation and promote healing.

Dosage Recommendations: For oral use, propolis can be consumed as tincture, extract, or capsules. Generally, 20-30 drops of propolis tincture taken 1-2 times daily or 500 mg of propolis extract taken 1-2 times daily are recommended for most therapeutic purposes. It is important to consult with a healthcare provider for personalized dosage recommendations.

Preparation Recipe: *Propolis Tincture:*

1. Ingredients:
   - 1 ounce raw propolis
   - 1 cup 70-95% ethanol (food-grade alcohol)
2. Preparation:
   - Break the raw propolis into small pieces and place it in a clean glass jar.
   - Pour the ethanol over the propolis pieces, ensuring they are fully submerged.
   - Seal the jar tightly and shake it gently.
   - Store the jar in a cool, dark place for 2-4 weeks, shaking it gently every few days.
   - After 2-4 weeks, strain the mixture through a fine mesh strainer or cheesecloth into a clean glass bottle, discarding the solids.
3. Serving:
   - Use a dropper to measure 20-30 drops of the propolis tincture and take it 1-2 times daily.
   - The tincture can be taken directly or added to water, tea, or juice.
   - Store the tincture in a cool, dark place.

Rhubarb (Rheum rhabarbarum)

Description: Rhubarb, scientifically known as Rheum rhabarbarum, is a perennial plant known for its large leaves and long, thick petioles (stalks) that are commonly used in culinary applications. While the stalks are edible and often used in desserts, the leaves are toxic due to their high oxalic acid content. Rhubarb has been used for centuries in traditional Chinese medicine for its medicinal properties, particularly its roots, which are known for their potent health benefits.

Antibiotic Properties: Rhubarb exhibits strong antibacterial properties primarily due to its high content of anthraquinones, such as emodin, aloe-emodin, and rhein. These compounds have demonstrated the ability to inhibit the growth of various pathogenic bacteria by disrupting their cell walls and metabolic processes. Studies have shown that rhubarb is effective against bacteria such as Staphylococcus aureus, Escherichia coli, and Salmonella spp. Additionally, rhubarb has antifungal and anti-inflammatory properties, further enhancing its antimicrobial efficacy.

Types of Infections Targeted: Rhubarb is effective in treating and preventing several internal infections:

- **Digestive Infections:** Rhubarb is particularly beneficial for treating gastrointestinal infections. Its antibacterial and anti-inflammatory properties help combat bacterial overgrowth and reduce symptoms of indigestion, bloating, and diarrhea.
- **Respiratory Infections:** Rhubarb can assist in alleviating symptoms of respiratory infections such as colds, bronchitis, and sinusitis. Its antimicrobial properties help eliminate pathogens and reduce inflammation.
- **Urinary Tract Infections (UTIs):** Rhubarb's diuretic and antibacterial properties make it useful in preventing and treating UTIs by promoting the elimination of bacteria and toxins from the urinary tract.

Dosage Recommendations: For oral use, rhubarb root can be consumed as a decoction, powder, or tincture. Generally, 0.5-2 grams of dried rhubarb root or 1-2 ml of rhubarb tincture taken 1-2 times daily are recommended for most therapeutic purposes.

It is important to consult with a healthcare provider for personalized dosage recommendations, especially for long-term use.

Preparation Recipe: *Rhubarb Root Decoction:*

1. **Ingredients:**
   - 1 teaspoon dried rhubarb root
   - 2 cups water
   - Honey or lemon (optional, for taste)
2. **Preparation:**
   - Place the dried rhubarb root in a saucepan with the water.
   - Bring the mixture to a boil, then reduce the heat and simmer for 20-30 minutes.
   - Remove from heat and let it cool slightly.
   - Strain the decoction into a cup.
3. **Serving:**
   - Add honey or lemon to taste, if desired.
   - Drink the decoction warm to benefit from its soothing and antibacterial properties.
   - Enjoy 1-2 cups daily to help prevent and treat various bacterial infections.

Rue (Ruta graveolens)

Description: Rue, scientifically known as Ruta graveolens, is a perennial herb native to the Mediterranean region. It is characterized by its blue-green leaves and small yellow flowers. Rue has been used since ancient times in traditional medicine for its various therapeutic properties. It has a strong, pungent aroma and a bitter taste, and it is often grown in gardens both for its ornamental value and its medicinal uses.

Antibiotic Properties: Rue possesses significant antibacterial properties due to its high content of alkaloids, flavonoids, and essential oils, including rutin, quercetin, and rutinose. These compounds have been shown to inhibit the growth of a variety of pathogenic bacteria by disrupting their cell walls and metabolic processes. Studies have demonstrated that rue is effective against bacteria such as Staphylococcus aureus, Escherichia coli, and Salmonella spp. Additionally, rue has antifungal and antiviral properties, which further enhance its antimicrobial profile.

Types of Infections Targeted: Rue is effective in treating and preventing several internal infections:

- **Respiratory Infections:** Rue can help alleviate symptoms of respiratory infections such as colds, bronchitis, and sinusitis. Its antibacterial and antiviral properties assist in eliminating pathogens and reducing inflammation.
- **Digestive Infections:** Rue aids in combating bacterial infections in the gastrointestinal tract, reducing symptoms of indigestion, bloating, and diarrhea.
- **Urinary Tract Infections (UTIs):** Rue's diuretic and antibacterial properties make it useful in preventing and treating UTIs by promoting the elimination of bacteria and toxins from the urinary tract.

Dosage Recommendations: For oral use, rue can be consumed as an infusion, tincture, or dried herb. Generally, 1-2 grams of dried rue or 1-2 ml of rue tincture taken 1-2 times daily are recommended for most therapeutic purposes. It is essential to consult with a healthcare provider for personalized dosage recommendations, especially for long-term use, as rue can be toxic in large amounts.

Preparation Recipe: *Rue Infusion:*

1. **Ingredients:**
    - 1 teaspoon dried rue leaves
    - 1 cup boiling water
    - Honey or lemon (optional, for taste)
2. **Preparation:**
    - Place the dried rue leaves in a tea infuser or teapot.
    - Pour the boiling water over the rue leaves.
    - Cover and let it steep for 10-15 minutes.
    - Strain the infusion into a cup.
3. **Serving:**
    - Add honey or lemon to taste, if desired.
    - Drink the infusion warm to benefit from its soothing and antibacterial properties.
    - Enjoy 1 cup daily to help prevent and treat various bacterial infections.

Wormwood (Artemisia absinthium)

Description: Wormwood, scientifically known as Artemisia absinthium, is a perennial herb native to Europe, North Africa, and Asia. It is characterized by its silvery-green leaves and small yellow flowers. Wormwood has a long history of use in traditional medicine and is well-known as a key ingredient in the alcoholic beverage absinthe. The herb is prized for its bitter taste and potent medicinal properties.

Antibiotic Properties: Wormwood possesses significant antibacterial properties due to its high content of sesquiterpene lactones, particularly absinthin and artemisinin. These compounds have demonstrated the ability to inhibit the growth of various pathogenic bacteria by disrupting their cell walls and metabolic processes. Studies have shown that wormwood is effective against bacteria such as Staphylococcus aureus, Escherichia coli, and Salmonella spp. Additionally, wormwood has antifungal, antiviral, and antiparasitic properties, further enhancing its antimicrobial profile.

Types of Infections Targeted: Wormwood is effective in treating and preventing several internal infections:

- **Digestive Infections:** Wormwood is particularly beneficial for treating gastrointestinal infections. Its antibacterial and antiparasitic properties help combat bacterial overgrowth and parasitic infections, reducing symptoms of indigestion, bloating, and diarrhea.
- **Respiratory Infections:** Wormwood can assist in alleviating symptoms of respiratory infections such as colds, bronchitis, and sinusitis. Its antimicrobial properties help eliminate pathogens and reduce inflammation.
- **Urinary Tract Infections (UTIs):** Wormwood's diuretic and antibacterial properties make it useful in preventing and treating UTIs by promoting the elimination of bacteria and toxins from the urinary tract.

Dosage Recommendations: For oral use, wormwood can be consumed as an infusion, tincture, or dried herb. Generally, 1-2 grams of dried wormwood or 1-2 ml of wormwood tincture taken 1-2 times daily are recommended for most therapeutic purposes. It is important to consult with a healthcare provider for personalized dosage recommendations, especially for long-term use, as wormwood can be toxic in large amounts.

Preparation Recipe: *Wormwood Infusion:*

1. **Ingredients:**
   - 1 teaspoon dried wormwood leaves
   - 1 cup boiling water
   - Honey or lemon (optional, for taste)
2. **Preparation:**
   - Place the dried wormwood leaves in a tea infuser or teapot.
   - Pour the boiling water over the wormwood leaves.
   - Cover and let it steep for 10-15 minutes.
   - Strain the infusion into a cup.
3. **Serving:**
   - Add honey or lemon to taste, if desired.
   - Drink the infusion warm to benefit from its soothing and antibacterial properties.

- Enjoy 1 cup daily to help prevent and treat various bacterial infections.

Dandelion (Taraxacum officinale)

Description: Dandelion, scientifically known as Taraxacum officinale, is a well-known perennial herbaceous plant that is native to Europe and Asia but now widespread across the globe. Recognizable by its bright yellow flowers and deeply toothed leaves, dandelion has been used in traditional medicine for centuries. Both the roots and the leaves are utilized for their medicinal properties, providing a variety of health benefits.

Antibiotic Properties: Dandelion exhibits antibacterial properties primarily due to its rich content of polyphenolic compounds, flavonoids, and sesquiterpene lactones. These compounds have demonstrated the ability to inhibit the growth of various pathogenic bacteria by disrupting their cell walls and interfering with their metabolic processes. Studies have shown that dandelion is effective against bacteria such as Staphylococcus aureus, Escherichia coli, and Pseudomonas aeruginosa. Additionally, dandelion has antioxidant and anti-inflammatory properties, which contribute to its overall therapeutic effects.

Types of Infections Targeted: Dandelion is effective in treating and preventing several internal infections:

- **Digestive Infections:** Dandelion is particularly beneficial for treating gastrointestinal infections. Its antibacterial properties help combat bacterial overgrowth in the digestive tract, reducing symptoms of indigestion, bloating, and constipation.
- **Respiratory Infections:** Dandelion can assist in alleviating symptoms of respiratory infections such as colds, bronchitis, and sinusitis. Its antimicrobial properties help eliminate pathogens and reduce inflammation.
- **Urinary Tract Infections (UTIs):** Dandelion's diuretic and antibacterial properties make it useful in preventing and treating UTIs by promoting the elimination of bacteria and toxins from the urinary tract.

Dosage Recommendations: For oral use, dandelion can be consumed as an infusion, tincture, or dried herb. Generally, 1-2 grams of dried dandelion root or 1-2 ml of dandelion tincture taken 1-2 times daily are recommended for most therapeutic purposes.

It is essential to consult with a healthcare provider for personalized dosage recommendations.

Preparation Recipe: *Dandelion Root Infusion:*

1. **Ingredients:**
   - 1 teaspoon dried dandelion root
   - 1 cup boiling water
   - Honey or lemon (optional, for taste)
2. **Preparation:**
   - Place the dried dandelion root in a tea infuser or teapot.
   - Pour the boiling water over the dandelion root.
   - Cover and let it steep for 10-15 minutes.
   - Strain the infusion into a cup.
3. **Serving:**
   - Add honey or lemon to taste, if desired.
   - Drink the infusion warm to benefit from its soothing and antibacterial properties.
   - Enjoy 1-2 cups daily to help prevent and treat various bacterial infections.

Bay Leaf (Laurus nobilis)

Description: Bay leaf, derived from the Laurus nobilis tree, is a fragrant, evergreen herb native to the Mediterranean region. The leaves are commonly used as a seasoning in cooking, known for their distinctive, slightly bitter flavor. Bay leaves have also been utilized in traditional medicine for their medicinal properties, including their antibacterial and anti-inflammatory effects.

Antibiotic Properties: Bay leaves exhibit significant antibacterial properties due to their high content of essential oils, including cineole, eugenol, and terpenes. These compounds have been shown to inhibit the growth of various pathogenic bacteria by disrupting their cell walls and metabolic processes. Studies have demonstrated that bay leaves are effective against bacteria such as Staphylococcus aureus, Escherichia coli, and Bacillus cereus. Additionally, bay leaves possess antifungal and antioxidant properties, which further enhance their antimicrobial profile.

Types of Infections Targeted: Bay leaves are effective in treating and preventing several internal infections:

- **Respiratory Infections:** Bay leaves can help alleviate symptoms of respiratory infections such as colds, bronchitis, and sinusitis. Their antibacterial and anti-inflammatory properties assist in eliminating pathogens and reducing inflammation.
- **Digestive Infections:** Bay leaves aid in combating bacterial infections in the gastrointestinal tract, reducing symptoms of indigestion, bloating, and flatulence.
- **Urinary Tract Infections (UTIs):** Bay leaves' diuretic and antibacterial properties make them useful in preventing and treating UTIs by promoting the elimination of bacteria and toxins from the urinary tract.

Dosage Recommendations: For oral use, bay leaves can be consumed as an infusion, powder, or in culinary dishes. Generally, 1-2 bay leaves or 1-2 grams of dried bay leaf powder taken 1-2 times daily are recommended for most therapeutic purposes. It is important to consult with a healthcare provider for personalized dosage recommendations.

Preparation Recipe: *Bay Leaf Infusion:*

1. **Ingredients:**
    - 1-2 dried bay leaves
    - 1 cup boiling water
    - Honey or lemon (optional, for taste)
2. **Preparation:**
    - Place the dried bay leaves in a tea infuser or teapot.
    - Pour the boiling water over the bay leaves.
    - Cover and let it steep for 10-15 minutes.
    - Strain the infusion into a cup.
3. **Serving:**
    - Add honey or lemon to taste, if desired.
    - Drink the infusion warm to benefit from its soothing and antibacterial properties.
    - Enjoy 1-2 cups daily to help prevent and treat various bacterial infections.

Fennel (Foeniculum vulgare)

Description: Fennel, scientifically known as Foeniculum vulgare, is a flowering plant species in the carrot family. Native to the Mediterranean, fennel has a long history of use in both culinary and medicinal traditions. The plant is known for its feathery leaves, yellow flowers, and distinct anise-like flavor. Both the bulb and seeds of fennel are used for their health benefits and aromatic qualities.

Antibiotic Properties: Fennel exhibits notable antibacterial properties due to its high content of essential oils, including anethole, fenchone, and estragole. These compounds have been shown to inhibit the growth of various pathogenic bacteria by disrupting their cell walls and metabolic processes. Research indicates that fennel is effective against bacteria such as Staphylococcus aureus, Escherichia coli, and Pseudomonas aeruginosa. Additionally, fennel has antifungal, antiviral, and anti-inflammatory properties, further enhancing its antimicrobial efficacy.

Types of Infections Targeted: Fennel is effective in treating and preventing several internal infections:

- **Digestive Infections:** Fennel is particularly beneficial for treating gastrointestinal infections. Its antibacterial and carminative properties help combat bacterial overgrowth, reducing symptoms of indigestion, bloating, and gas.
- **Respiratory Infections:** Fennel can assist in alleviating symptoms of respiratory infections such as colds, bronchitis, and sinusitis. Its antimicrobial properties help eliminate pathogens and reduce inflammation.
- **Urinary Tract Infections (UTIs):** Fennel's diuretic and antibacterial properties make it useful in preventing and treating UTIs by promoting the elimination of bacteria and toxins from the urinary tract.

Dosage Recommendations: For oral use, fennel seeds can be consumed as an infusion, tincture, or dried herb. Generally, 1-2 grams of dried fennel seeds or 1-2 ml of fennel tincture taken 1-2 times daily are recommended for most therapeutic purposes. It is essential to consult with a healthcare provider for personalized dosage recommendations.

Preparation Recipe: *Fennel Seed Infusion:*

1. **Ingredients:**
   - 1 teaspoon dried fennel seeds
   - 1 cup boiling water
   - Honey or lemon (optional, for taste)
2. **Preparation:**
   - Place the dried fennel seeds in a tea infuser or teapot.
   - Pour the boiling water over the fennel seeds.
   - Cover and let it steep for 10-15 minutes.
   - Strain the infusion into a cup.
3. **Serving:**
   - Add honey or lemon to taste, if desired.
   - Drink the infusion warm to benefit from its soothing and antibacterial properties.
   - Enjoy 1-2 cups daily to help prevent and treat various bacterial infections.

Garlic Chives (Allium tuberosum)

Description: Garlic chives, scientifically known as Allium tuberosum, are a perennial herb native to East Asia. Also known as Chinese chives, these plants are characterized by their flat, grass-like leaves and small, white star-shaped flowers. Garlic chives have a mild garlic flavor and are commonly used in culinary applications. They are also valued for their medicinal properties, which have been utilized in traditional medicine for centuries.

Antibiotic Properties: Garlic chives possess significant antibacterial properties due to their high content of sulfur compounds, including allicin and alliin. These compounds are known for their ability to inhibit the growth of various pathogenic bacteria by disrupting their cell walls and interfering with their metabolic processes. Studies have shown that garlic chives are effective against bacteria such as Staphylococcus aureus, Escherichia coli, and Salmonella spp. Additionally, garlic chives have antifungal and antiviral properties, which further enhance their antimicrobial profile.

Types of Infections Targeted: Garlic chives are effective in treating and preventing several internal infections:

- **Digestive Infections:** Garlic chives are particularly beneficial for treating gastrointestinal infections. Their antibacterial properties help combat bacterial overgrowth, reducing symptoms of indigestion, bloating, and diarrhea.
- **Respiratory Infections:** Garlic chives can assist in alleviating symptoms of respiratory infections such as colds, bronchitis, and sinusitis. Their antimicrobial properties help eliminate pathogens and reduce inflammation.
- **Urinary Tract Infections (UTIs):** Garlic chives' diuretic and antibacterial properties make them useful in preventing and treating UTIs by promoting the elimination of bacteria and toxins from the urinary tract.

Dosage Recommendations: For oral use, garlic chives can be consumed fresh, as an infusion, or in culinary dishes. Generally, 1-2 grams of fresh garlic chives or 1-2 ml of garlic chive juice taken 1-2 times daily are recommended for most therapeutic purposes.

It is essential to consult with a healthcare provider for personalized dosage recommendations.

Preparation Recipe: *Garlic Chive Infusion:*

1. **Ingredients:**
    o   1 tablespoon fresh garlic chives, chopped
    o   1 cup boiling water
    o   Honey or lemon (optional, for taste)
2. **Preparation:**
    o   Place the chopped garlic chives in a tea infuser or teapot.
    o   Pour the boiling water over the garlic chives.
    o   Cover and let it steep for 10-15 minutes.
    o   Strain the infusion into a cup.
3. **Serving:**
    o   Add honey or lemon to taste, if desired.
    o   Drink the infusion warm to benefit from its soothing and antibacterial properties.
    o   Enjoy 1-2 cups daily to help prevent and treat various bacterial infections.

Barberry (Berberis vulgaris)

Description: Barberry, scientifically known as Berberis vulgaris, is a shrub native to Europe and parts of Asia. The plant is recognized for its bright red berries, yellow flowers, and thorny branches. Barberry has been used in traditional medicine for centuries, particularly for its medicinal bark, roots, and berries. The key active compound in barberry is berberine, which is responsible for its various health benefits.

Antibiotic Properties: Barberry exhibits potent antibacterial properties primarily due to its high content of berberine. Berberine is an alkaloid that has been shown to inhibit the growth of various pathogenic bacteria by disrupting their cell walls, interfering with their protein synthesis, and inhibiting their enzyme activity. Studies have demonstrated that barberry is effective against bacteria such as Staphylococcus aureus, Escherichia coli, and Salmonella spp. Additionally, barberry possesses antifungal, antiviral, and anti-inflammatory properties, further enhancing its antimicrobial profile.

Types of Infections Targeted: Barberry is effective in treating and preventing several internal infections:

- **Digestive Infections:** Barberry is particularly beneficial for treating gastrointestinal infections. Its antibacterial properties help combat bacterial overgrowth in the digestive tract, reducing symptoms of indigestion, diarrhea, and dysentery.
- **Respiratory Infections:** Barberry can assist in alleviating symptoms of respiratory infections such as colds, bronchitis, and sinusitis. Its antimicrobial properties help eliminate pathogens and reduce inflammation.
- **Urinary Tract Infections (UTIs):** Barberry's diuretic and antibacterial properties make it useful in preventing and treating UTIs by promoting the elimination of bacteria and toxins from the urinary tract.

Dosage Recommendations: For oral use, barberry can be consumed as an infusion, tincture, or extract. Generally, 1-2 grams of dried barberry root or 1-2 ml of barberry tincture taken 1-2 times daily are recommended for most therapeutic purposes.

It is essential to consult with a healthcare provider for personalized dosage recommendations.

Preparation Recipe: *Barberry Root Infusion:*

1. **Ingredients:**
   - 1 teaspoon dried barberry root
   - 1 cup boiling water
   - Honey or lemon (optional, for taste)
2. **Preparation:**
   - Place the dried barberry root in a tea infuser or teapot.
   - Pour the boiling water over the barberry root.
   - Cover and let it steep for 10-15 minutes.
   - Strain the infusion into a cup.
3. **Serving:**
   - Add honey or lemon to taste, if desired.
   - Drink the infusion warm to benefit from its soothing and antibacterial properties.
   - Enjoy 1-2 cups daily to help prevent and treat various bacterial infections.

Legal Disclaimer

The information provided in "Nature's Apothecary: Quick Reference Guide to Oral Antibiotics" is intended for educational and informational purposes only. It is not intended as a substitute for professional medical advice, diagnosis, or treatment. Always seek the advice of your physician or other qualified health providers with any questions you may have regarding a medical condition. Never disregard professional medical advice or delay in seeking it because of something you have read in this book.

The authors and publishers of this book are not liable for any adverse effects or consequences resulting from the use of any suggestions, preparations, or procedures described in this book. The use of any information provided in this book is solely at your own risk.

Herbal remedies and supplements are not regulated by the Food and Drug Administration (FDA) and may have different effects on different individuals. It is important to conduct your own research and consult with a healthcare provider before using any new herb or supplement, especially if you are pregnant, nursing, have a medical condition, or are taking any medication.

This book does not provide medical, legal, or other professional advice. The authors and publishers do not assume any responsibility or liability for the accuracy, completeness, or usefulness of the information contained in this book. The inclusion of any herb or remedy in this book does not imply endorsement by the authors or publishers.

By using this book, you acknowledge and agree to the terms of this disclaimer.

Meet the Author

Hey everyone, just wanted to invite everyone to join me on my social pages. Links below!

Facebook Page....Luna Parnell's Written Works

Patreon page.... patreon.com/Lunastreasures